ALKALINE DIET

Follow the Natural Action Plan and Find Out How These High Alkaline Foods Will Prolong Your Life, Helping You Purify and Treat Your Body and Lose Weight, Without Being a Dieting Pro (Part 1)

By
Chelsea Morris

© Copyright 2020 - All rights reserved.

declared or implied. Readers acknowledge that the author is not engaging in the rendering of legal, financial, medical or professional advice. The content within this book has been derived from various sources. Please consult a licensed professional before attempting any techniques outlined in this book.

By reading this document, the reader agrees that under no circumstances is the author responsible for any losses, direct or indirect, which are incurred as a result of the use of information contained within this document, including, but not limited to, — errors, omissions, or inaccuracies.

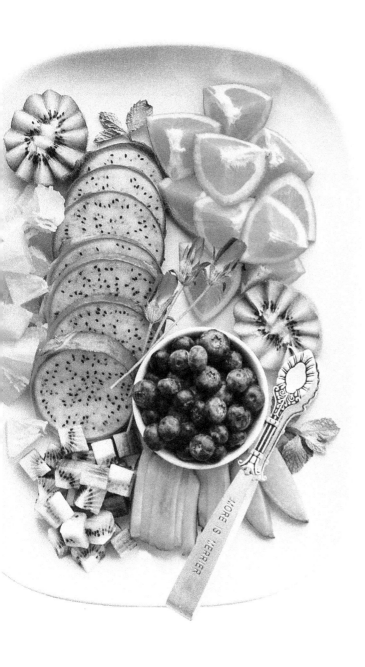

Table of Contents

Introduction

I want to thank you and congratulate you for buying the book, *"Alkaline Diet"*

This book contains information on Alkaline diet. Do you an holistic approach to well-being and healthy life? Well, alkaline diet is the way to go. It is a simple diet that will give a natural healthy body which is everyone's desire.

The benefits of the diet are many and great for you. Irrespective of the age you have and your level of health, if you follow the on the information found in this book, you will enjoy the immense benefits of this amazing diet and you will not want to turn back from it.

The diet is a powerful anti-aging program that will transform you from the inside out. Some of its benefits improved skin tone, hair luster, increased vitality, and weight loss. It makes your immune stronger, improved brain functions and bones stronger

Thanks for downloading this book. It's my firm belief that it will provide you with all the answers to your questions

Chapter 1:
Alkaline Diet Explained

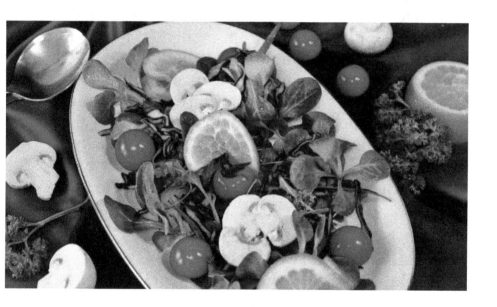

What is Alkaline Diet?

The alkaline diet is a prescription for health designed to help pull your body out of its acidic state by balancing your acid/alkaline intake. It identifies the acid-forming or acidic food as being responsible for obstructing the healthy rate of metabolism and disrupting an optimal pH environment in the body. The alkaline diet simply restricts the acidic food and promotes the use of more alkaline food. The diet is constituted by measuring the pH values of the ingredients, and then they are added to the meal.

What is pH?

pH stands for potential of hydrogen. It is the scale which determines the acidity or alkalinity of a substance. The range of the pH scale is 0-14. 7 is the neutral point in the scale. A higher number mean that highly alkaline and a lower number means that the food is acidic. The most appropriate human body pH is 7.3. It is therefore good to eat a lot of alkaline food to maintain this level. The levels of pH id different in the human body. The most acidic part is the stomach. This is because it has acids which help in digestion of food.

How Alkaline Diet Works

It's simple – the goal of the alkaline diet is to make and keep the acid-alkaline balance in your organism. It does this by decreasing the amount of acid you consume, and it helps you lose weight by making the acidic components in your fat cells convert into energy. The nutrition experts suggest that your diet should contain 80 percent of vegetables and others alkaline-promoting foods. As you can see, you are only allowed 20 percent of highly acidic foods, such as meat, when you start this way of nutrition.

That ration of 80:20 will help your organism keep its pH balance. The experts noticed that it doesn't only help you lose weight, but it helps you burn fat in those parts where you hate it the most – on your belly and your hips.

Advantages of the Alkaline Diet
More energy

Cells must function well in order for the body to produce and use energy well. Acidity interferes with proper cellular processes and reduces energy levels. By going alkaline, the cells can function better. More energy will be produced and the other cells will have more to use for their own functions. This will result to higher energy levels.

Better gum and dental health

If the body is too acidic, the oral cavity is also acidic. Acidity will cause the dental enamel to erode, which will promote the formation of dental carries, plaques and cavities. This is also among the leading causes of bad breath. The acidic environment in the mouth promotes the overgrowth of bacteria. This will cause several oral health problems such as various gum diseases. This will also increase the risk for tooth decay. Most people notice improvement in their breath and overall dental health once they go on an alkaline diet.

Better immunity

When the various cells in the body are healthy, the immune system functions better. The integrity of the cells is great. Cellular integrity protects the cells from infections. The pathogens will find it difficult to enter and cause trouble. If the pH in the body is low (acidic), the cells will find it hard to keep their structures intact. This will allow toxins and pathogens to easily enter and cause more damage. These pathogens and toxins can easily get inside the cells and alter it. This will stimulate the development of health problems. Cancer, for instance, starts off this way. This is also a major reason why some people more frequently get colds and other infections compared to those who follow the alkaline diet.

Reduction in inflammation and pain

Magnesium is an important mineral in the body. It also has a vital role in maintaining the body's pH balance. If the body becomes acidic, the cells will release their magnesium stores to help in neutralizing the acidity. The more acidic the body, the more magnesium is required to counter its effects. This may be ideal but magnesium does not only function for acid neutralizing. The body has so many other uses for magnesium. Using a lot for acid neutralizing can seriously deplete the resources for the other tissues and cellular processes to use.

One of the major tissues affected is the joint. Low magnesium in the body is one of the factors that cause joint diseases and inflammatory conditions. Also, inflammation in the other tissues in the body is also attributed to low magnesium stores. Eating alkaline foods that are also rich in magnesium can replenish the resources and have more for the cells to use.

It strengthens the Neurons

When neurological processes are restored and protected, you get to protect yourself from Alzheimer's Disease and memory loss. Degenerative diseases could also be prevented.

This happens because alkaline foods also contain L -Theanine, an amino acid that promotes better neurological health—and not a lot of food products are able to do this.

Weight Control

This is a culmination of all the positive effects of alkalinity in the body. The cells function better, so that energy is better distributed. Fats are used properly and the body has enough energy. This will reduce cravings and hunger cues. That means reduction in the frequency of hunger cues and better appetite control. Fats and energy are also burned much better, reducing the risk of accumulating more fats that contribute to weight gain.

Preventing Stomach Upset

Thermogenesis, the term given to fat to energy conversion, is increased by at least 8 to 10 % when someone uses alkaline foods in his daily diet. This not only burns fat, but also regulates the digestive process.

Alkaline foods also reduce intestinal gas, and could also prevent certain diseases from happening, such as ulcers, ulcerative colitis, and Chron's Disease.

Slower Aging Process

The aging process is driven by the damage to cells. When cells easily degrade and repair is slow, the aging process is accelerated. If the cells are able to repair damage efficiently and at a faster rate, the aging process slows down. In an acidic environment, the cells get easily damaged and at a much faster rate. Repair is slowed in acidic pH. In an alkaline environment, cells do not get as much damage and when any injury gets repaired sooner.

Also, the aging process is accelerated due to oxidative stress. This is caused by the accumulation of free radicals and toxins that eat away at the cells. Acidic pH in the body supports oxidative stress. Alkaline pH helps in reducing the toxin load and oxidative stress. These promote younger-looking, healthier cells that give a younger appearance.

Perfect for Athletes

This is mainly because they know that if they eat too much fat, their bodies would suffer, and their hearts would grow weaker—and that's never a good thing because they live such active lives. Even superstars such as LeBron James have actually pledged allegiance to the low carb diet—so why won't you?

More so, when you adhere to these diets, it would be easy for your body to turn nutrients into ketogenic energy. When you have ketones in your system, you get to perk yourself up, and you get to have enough energy to get through the day—and help you out with whatever it is that you have to do!

Plus, when it comes to weight loss, you really cannot expect that you'd lose weigh if you keep on eating too much fats and carbohydrates. It's just not right, and won't work well with what you have in mind. Since regular exercise is said to work best with the Alkaline Diets, you can keep in mind that you could make it a part of your life—so you could be sure that the diet would really work.

Avoiding Chronic Inflammation

Chronic inflammation is the reason why so many diseases happen. These diseases include Type 2 Diabetes, Heart Problems, and Cancer. This so happens because grains are—you guessed it—inflammatory. While you may not see the effects right away, in time, you'd notice how your body would disintegrate, and how you'd feel like you're no longer in shape, and that your health is on the downlow. When you keep on eating grains, you're just fueling up the problem instead of working on ways to solve it.

Staying away from Auto-Immune Diseases

Take a look at it this way: Gliadin, also known as the worst kind of gluten, is actually responsible for affecting the pancreas, thyroids, and the entire immune system by means of releasing antibodies that aren't meant to get out yet. When these antibodies go out, auto-immune diseases come into play and one may be afflicted with diseases such as Hashimoto's Disease, type 1 diabetes, and hypothyroidism, among others.

Incidentally, research has it that Alzheimer's Disease is often triggered by high-grain diets. It releasers blockers in the brain that could break mental processes down, and therefore lead to the deterioration of the brain.

Develop a Healthy Gut

Doctors believe that the state of your gut could affect the state of your brain. After all, when you're hungry, you tend to make decisions that are not well thought out.

As you can see, your gut is in charge of a lot of things in your body—which you often fail to see in your daily life. These things include the way you utilize fat and carbohydrates; nutrient absorption; being satiated; vitamin and neurotransmitter production; inflammation; detoxification, and immunity against diseases, amongst others.

This is also because of the vagus nerve, found in the gut, which is the longest of the 12 cranial nerves. This is the main channel between your digestive system, and your nerve cells that send signals to the brain.

In short, it would be wrong for you not to take care of your gut because it would be like a way of putting your own health in danger. Why? Well, because if the given processes above does not work right, you might be afflicted with certain medical conditions, such as dementia, diabetes, allergies, cancer, ADHD, asthma, and other chronic health problems.

Not only that, the clarity of your thoughts, and the way you feel are also affected. When you don't eat what's right for you, you might be afflicted with anxiety, depression, or other problems that won't make life easy for you.

When your gut is healthy, your brain gets to make more serotonin—the hormone that keeps you happy, and keeps your sanity in check—one that not even the best anti-depressants could give out too much, and this is why you have to make sure that you start eating right.

Avoid Vitamin-D Deficiency

Even if you consume Vitamin D, it actually depletes inside the body pretty fast, and acid makes depletion even faster. More so, WGA, or Wheat Germ Agglutinin also causes bacterial growth that kills Vitamin D, and damages the gut—and could do much worse to your body in the future.

Prevention of Dehydration

Unlike coffee and soda, alkaline food makes an amazing drink because it keeps the body hydrated, and makes sure that dehydration is prevented. Alkaline food has moisture, as mentioned in an earlier chapter, which means that it actually has water, unlike other flavored or carbonated drinks.

Feeling So Much Better

It sounds cheesy, sure, but the thing is when you adhere to this diet combination, it's like you're giving yourself the chance to feel good again.

These days, people go through a lot of things. Their lives—possibly yours, too—could turn nasty in just a second, and it would be even harder if they don't take care of their health. So, as early as now, you should consider this book a chance for you to reverse your health—for the better, of course!

Chapter 2:
Alkaline or Acid?

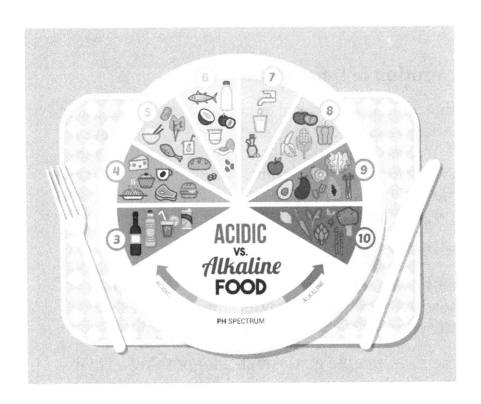

What Alkaline/Acid Mean

Alkaline means having a pH scale of 7.1 to 14 on the pH scale. Basically, if any food falls within this range, it can be said to be alkaline.

Acidic means having a pH scale of 0 to 6.99 on the pH scale. Any food said to acidic falls within range.

Alkaline- and Acid-Forming Foods

While many foods obviously fall into an acid or alkaline category, others aren't quite as evident at first glance. Take a lemon, for example. You know a lemon tastes tart, so it must clearly be acidic, right? While the nature of a lemon is acidic, once it is metabolized by the body, it has an alkalizing effect. Foods that are acidic in nature are not always acid forming once they are consumed. Many acidic foods like citrus, kefir, and sauerkraut are healing and alkalizing. To add to the confusion, numerous charts on acidifying and alkalizing foods simply use the words "acid foods" and "alkaline foods," which really doesn't give an accurate picture.

According to the journal *Seminars in Dialysis*, to precisely forecast the base or acid present in a particular food, scientists worked long and hard and came up with a technique that takes into account the food's nutrient composition and, in layman's terms, can determine what the true base or acid content on the body is. Thus, was born the potential renal acid load (PRAL) scale. A negative score means the diet is alkaline/basic. Acidic foods have positive scores. For neutral food, the score is 0. If you add the PRAL values for all the foods you eat in a day, you get the net acid or alkaline load. While it isn't necessary to micromanage your diet to get the lowest PRAL values, it may be interesting to calculate the PRAL values of your normal diet.

Signs of Being Too Acidic

Weight gain – a body that has high acid levels can create additional insulin and store extra amounts of fat. The problem is that your body can't process the excess acid by itself. Instead, it just pushes it back into the fat cells and stores it. Additionally, highly acidic organisms have trouble to burn calories efficiently, so if you feel your body is not losing weight at the pace it should that might be the reason.

Bone weakness – are your bones prone to fractures? That might happen because you have an overly acidic body. If you take a lot of acids, your organism will take potassium from your bones to regulate it and leave you with weaker bones. In the long-term, that can also lead to developing osteoporosis. If you know anyone suffering from this disease, then you surely noticed that their nutrition changed ever since they were diagnosed. That is because doctor's advice patients with osteoporosis to limit the intake of acid-promoting foods.

Your teeth are sensitive - if you noticed tooth decay, the cause behind it could be acid. In a study published in the International Journal of Chemical Applications and Engineering, tooth enamel erosion is correlated with overly acidic bodies. The best way to check the sensitiveness of your teeth is to eat hot or cold foods. If a tooth reacts, the chances are there is a cavity on it.

Sleep deprivations – high levels of acid cause sleep disorders with some people. This is also related to levels of potassium, which can cause insomnia.

Other health problems acidosis may cause include stiff neck, sciatica, shortness of breath and other respiratory problems, arrhythmias and other heart problems, diabetes, kidney infections, premature aging, joint pain, and even allergies. That is why it's important to monitor your pH levels and keep them in order.

How to Check Acidic Levels

The first thing you need to know is that tracking pH levels is easy and inexpensive. Most people give up believing that it's hard to test their acidic levels, but it's simple, and it won't take much of your time, considering that each test takes up to 30 seconds. You will need a pH test strip to check your acidic levels. You can get them in a drug store nearby, and they are relatively cheap. If you want to track how your pH levels vary regularly, you will also need a notebook or something where you will write your results.

Let's be clear on one thing – a single test won't prove anything. I recommend that you track your pH for at least one month. That way you will have relevant results, and you will have the opportunity to see the effect of your nutrition choices.

These are steps you need to take when measuring your pH:

Morning Saliva Test

After you wake up, use a dual pH test strip to check your saliva. Make sure not to brush your teeth, drink any water, or eat any food. You want it to be as soon as you open your eyes.

You do this test by simply using your saliva to lick and wet the end of the test strip. There's an even more accurate way – use a spoon. Spit your saliva onto it, and then dip the test strip into the spoon. Make sure to wait 15-20 seconds for the results. The color of the strip will change, and that is when you should check out the pH number and write it down. Experts believe that the best level of pH upon waking up is anywhere between 6.8 and 7.2.

Morning Urine Test

The next step you need to take is to test your urine after waking up. Note that this should be the very first urine of that day. That way you can measure the urine that you kept in your bladder overnight. Just put the test strip in the urine when it's mid-stream. Shake off all the excess fluid and wait for the results for about 15 seconds. When the color changes, write down the pH level the strip shows.

Just like the morning saliva test, your level should vary between 6.8 and 7.2. I know that I mentioned that is not the ideal pH level, but keep in mind that you stored the acids overnight, so it's only normal for your body to be a bit more acidic in the morning.

You shouldn't worry if your results are over 7.2. That means your body is alkaline and your way of eating does the job of keeping your pH in order. The problem occurs if your pH level is lower than 6.8. That is a sign that you need to make some changes to your nutrition, reduce acid and add more alkaline buffers. You can do that by adding organic greens, and alkaline water to your diet, but we will talk about that later.

The morning tests of your saliva and urine will show you how efficient your digestive system was with dealing with what you ate and drank during the previous day/evening. You should notice these numbers come up with time once you start an alkaline diet.

Second Urine Test

After you tested the first urine, you also need to test your second urine on a particular day. If it is by any means possible, you should do this before you have breakfast (or consuming any food). Naturally, you can take a green drink or water in the meantime. The goal is to perform a post-hydration test of your urine. Conduct the test the same way you did the first one, notice the pH number and write it down.

The first urine will help you expel the metabolic acids your organism kept in your bladder overnight. That is why the second test should show a higher number, ideally between 7.2 and 7.4.

Keep Track for At Least One Month

You should calculate your average pH number based on two urine tests you conducted. That will be the number you will use for that day.

Once you start an alkaline diet, you can also conduct the test during the day to see how your organism reacts. For example, use a test strip to measure your pH level between two meals. Don't be surprised if your pH levels are a bit higher right after you ate. The ideal range is between 7.2 and 7.4, but anywhere up to 8.4 is acceptable if you did the test just after you finished the meal.

You can also check your acidic levels right after you ate something with high alkaline levels, such as green drink, almond butter, water with lemon, mineral salts, etc.). During the day, your pH number should go a bit up from the initial morning test. If it goes down or stays the same, that's a sign that you lack mineral reserves and that your organism is eating its resources to fight the excess amount of acid.

Dangers of Being Too Acidic

Some of the effects of eating consuming too much acidic foods include;

- Sensitive gums
- Mood swings
- Acne
- Depression
- Brittle hair and nails
- Listlessness
- Dry skin
- Headaches
- Acidosis
- pH imbalance

Chapter 3:
Foods to Eat/Avoid

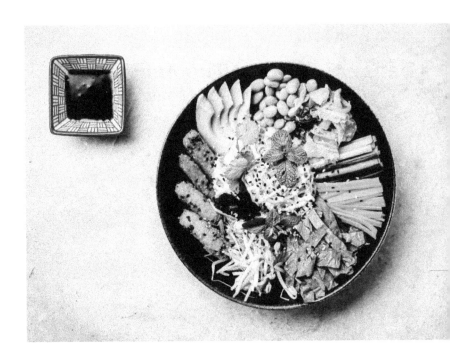

Foods to Eat

Root Vegetables

These plants fall into that category of food you can eat as much as you like when you are on the alkaline diet. You see, root vegetables contain more minerals than most of the other veggies, which is why you should consume them as often as possible. My recommendation is to eat all types of radish (white, red, black), as well as horseradish. You can also eat carrots, beets, turnips, and rutabaga. The best way to prepare root veggies is by just steaming them for about 15 minutes. Their biggest advantage aside from securing you a lot of minerals is that you will feel full after eating them.

Cruciferous Vegetables

Another type of veggies you can freely consume. Cruciferous vegetables include cabbage, broccoli, Brussels sprouts, and cauliflower. Feel free to consume them with a homemade healthy pesto sauce.

Leafy Greens

The alkaline diet requires you to eat a lot of vegetables, so it's not strange that we are continuing our list of veggies with leafy greens. Swiss chard, spinach, kale, and turnip greens all should find their way to your list. I would like to single out spinach because it has a high amount of vitamin K, as well as minerals, fiber, and antioxidants that can improve your digestive system.

Garlic

Garlic also needs to be singled down because it can be considered as a miracle food. Various diets recommend garlic and the alkaline way of nutrition is not different. There are good reasons for that since garlic helps your immune and cardiovascular systems, lowers your blood pressure, and cleanses your liver.

Cayenne Peppers

Cayenne peppers are also among the alkaline-promoting foods. It is incredibly rich in vitamin A and other antibacterial properties, which is crucial for fighting various diseases and stress. It also contains enzymes that improve your body's endocrine function.

Lemon

Your parents undoubtedly told you how lemon is great for fighting colds and flu. These are not just stories as they are completely right. Lemons not only fight viruses, but it also acts as an excellent disinfectant for healing wounds. It also helps you detoxify your organism and energizes your liver.

As you can see, vegetables are the most important part of your nutrition in the alkaline diet.

I tried to emphasize those that are highly alkaline to help you efficiently increase your pH levels. However, that doesn't mean that you shouldn't eat other veggies, too.

Foods to Avoid
Processed Foods and Other High-Sodium Foods

Processed foods are unhealthy for your organism. They contain high levels of sodium chloride, also known as table salt. Processed foods constrict your blood vessels and belong to the category of acid-promoting food. If you like salt, go with sea salt or Himalayan salt.

Conventional Meats and Cold Cuts

In one word, you should avoid all overly-processed meats. It is recommended that the meat you eat is grass-fed and, even in that case, you should make sure to limit its intake according to the 80/20 ratio we mentioned for the alkaline diet.

You can also eliminate meat from your nutrition completely and still secure enough nutrients to keep recommended pH levels.

Oats and Other Whole-Wheat Products

Grains are one of the main reasons why your body is overly acidic. It doesn't matter if the grains are whole or not, it will contribute to the acid levels in your organism. Make sure to avoid corn flakes and other processed cereals.

Eggs and Milk

Food rich in calcium can cause osteoporosis because of the acid they create in the body.

We already talked about how the body robs your bones of calcium to get the pH level in balance. Eggs and milk elevate your acidity, so it might be best to avoid them.

Coffee and Alcohol

All types of alcohol contribute to acidity in your body, so you should steer clear of it at all times. It's similar to coffee and other caffeinated drinks, considering that they are also among the acid-promoting drinks. High caffeine intake is related to higher level of acid in numerous studies.

Aside from making sure which food to avoid, you should also make sure to avoid artificial sweeteners, food preservatives, and coloring, as well as overusing antibiotics or using drugs at all. You should also make sure always to have time to properly chew your food as it can help decrease the acidity of your body.

•

Chapter 4:
Frequently Asked Questions

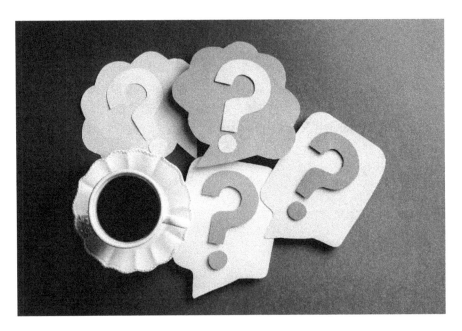

Q: Can alkaline foods also prevent Alzheimer's Disease?

According to a couple of studies done over the years, especially those performed by the University of Newcastle, Alkaline Foods actually improves memory, and when one's memory is good, Alzheimer's Disease could be prevented in the long run.

This is because alkaline foods affect the cholinergic system of the brain, which, when damaged, contributes to the risk of getting Alzheimer's in the future. Alkaline foods hydrolyze the enzymes that could destroy the said system, and therefore get to protect the brain from further damage.

Also, studies have shown that alkaline food contains the same elements as pharmaceutical products do—minus the side effects, and while working for a long period of time. This means that the effects will not only be prevalent today, but as long as one has alkaline foods in his diet.

Q: Is it true that alkaline foods are good for healthy aging?

Yes, absolutely.

Since alkaline foods restore the skin's elasticity due to its antioxidant content, healthy aging is promoted. Take for example those in countries that naturally drink alkaline foods (i.e., Japan)—you can see that they age gracefully, compared to those who just drink it occasionally, and whose diets are mostly made up of preservatives.

Research also has it that those who drink alkaline foods live longer—without having to worry about diseases that old age could bring.

Q: Can the quality of water affect the quality of alkaline foods?

Yes, it could.

You know, alkaline foods actually taste better when polyphenols and caffeine meet each other, and work together—and this only happens when you get to brew alkaline foods properly, and not in overcooked or over boiled water.

Overcooked water dampens the taste of the alkaline foods. When it's no longer palatable, you may feel like you shouldn't add it in your diet anymore—and that's what you have to prevent from happening.

Q: Can alkaline foods prevent stroke?

When eaten regularly, yes, there is a chance.

This is because alkaline foods contain polyphenols and antioxidants that the body easily absorbs to protect itself from free radicals that may bring forth stroke and cancer. While doing so, it also clears the digestive tract, and could also protect one from most degenerative diseases, too.

Q: Are alkaline foods bad for pregnant women?

First and foremost, this is just a myth.

Studies show that consuming alkaline foods has no effects to either the pregnant and lactating mother, or to her child, whether through growth retention, or miscarriages. There are also no effects of alkaline foods caffeine on child development and mental processes.

However, when one already has an aversion to alkaline foods, and often suffers from indigestion when consuming caffeine, it's best to consult the doctor first before drinking alkaline foods. It's also best to eat a healthy diet and exercise regularly even when one is pregnant, so that birth will be easy, and so the woman would be able to maintain good health while taking care of her child, as well.

A pregnant woman could drink up to 3 to 4 cups of alkaline foods each day, but has to refrain from coffee as it may bring forth palpitations.

Q: Are alkaline foods really good for my immune system?

Yes, especially when you take it regularly. This is because it boosts the body's capability to bring infection down, and could also track germs better— so the immune system could drive them away from the body.

Q: It's said that alkaline food blocks iron absorption. Is this true?

Absolutely not. Dietary iron has two forms, which are non-heme iron (plant iron), and heme iron (animal iron). When you consume alkaline foods, your body still gets to absorb at least 15 to 35% of heme, and 25% of non-heme iron—which means you'd get the amazing dietary benefits that they bring.

It's also easy to absorb polyphenols and ascorbic acid with the help of alkaline foods, as well.

Q: What makes the Flat Alkaline Foods Belly Diet healthy? What are the nutrients that one could get from alkaline foods?

As there are various kinds of alkaline food, you can expect that nutritional content varies, too. But mostly, you can expect that you'll get the following:

Sodium. Sodium prevents hypertension.

Protein. Protein is one of the most important nutrients that the body needs to function well. You can get at least 2% or more of it from one cup of alkaline foods.

Potassium. Potassium helps cells do their job properly. Alkaline foods contain a lot of potassium.

Magnesium. Magnesium is essential for the strength and growth of the human body, and could also prevent tissue breakage.

Lipids. Lipids are good kinds of fat that are mostly mixed with protein and could help hair become stronger.

Fluorine. Fluorine helps make teeth stronger.

Carbohydrates. Alkaline foods contain around 4 to 5% of carbohydrates—so you could omit rice and other grains from your diet.

Calcium and Phosphorous. These are both needed for bones to grow strong. Teeth could benefit from them, too.

Also, you could expect that with the help of alkaline foods, you will get to fill your dietary needs by getting:

- 6% Vitamin B6
- 25% Vitamin B2
- 9% Vitamin B1
- 10% Zinc
- 16% Calcium

Around 50% of flavonoids and anti-oxidants.

In short, if you want to live a healthy life, you definitely should add alkaline foods in your diet.

Chapter 5:
The Alkaline Lifestyle

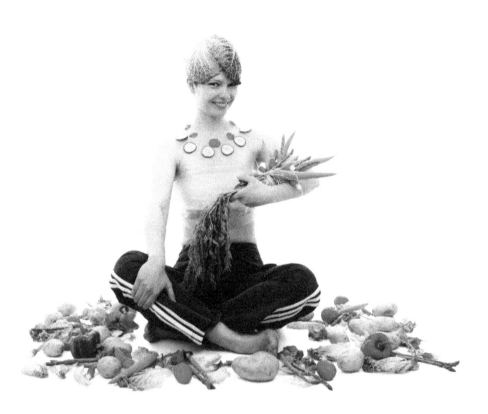

Guideline for Eating Alkaline Diet

- Concentrate on whole foods like whole grains, seeds, beans, spices, nuts, vegetables, fruits and root crops.

- Consume less of pasta, fish, essential fats and meat.
- Avoid white flour, caffeine, artificial/processed foods and white sugar.
- Take alkalizing drinks like whole lemon or lime juice, ginger root and spring water.
- Dress your salads and also use fats of high quality like avocado oil, olive oil and coconut oil.

Tips to Become More Alkaline

Do breathing exercises regularly – three times a day is the frequency for deep breathing exercises. Deep breathing will help you get rid of carbon dioxide, which is the most damaging acid in your organism. Believe it or not, carbon dioxide is 115 times more acidic than all the others acids in your body TOGETHER.

Stay hydrated – I once again mention the importance of staying hydrated. Yes, it's that important! Please note that coffee doesn't count. You can take a big glass of water (8 ounces) with one-half of lemon juice and two tablespoons of apple cider vinegar in the morning. Also, make sure to drink enough water each day. A recommended amount is half your body weight in ounces. For example, if you weigh 170 lbs. You need to consume 85 oz. of water every day.

Drink smoothies – a great way to get some alkaline-promoting foods in your body is to make yourself a fresh green smoothie. The winning combination should be kale or spinach, a small number of berries or banana and healthy fats such as chia seeds, raw almond butter, and coconut oil.

Proper Digestion

Proper digestion is essential for every diet, and it is crucial for the alkaline way of nutrition. After eating highly acidic foods for a while, they affect your digestive system by clogging it. Bacteria, yeast, candida, and mycotoxins all find their way to your gastrointestinal tract, meaning that your organism produces more waste and becomes more acidic. Irritable bowel syndrome is only one of the things that yeasts and bacteria can cause. Aside from causing you problems, a much bigger worry is that your organism can only use a small portion of all those nutrients you have been consuming. Yeasts and other undigested matters coat the walls of your intestines and prevent nutrients from entering and your body to absorb them. That is why it is incredibly important to cleanse your digestive system and allow it to function properly. That means that you will improve your nutrients absorption and, therefore, your diet results through no extra work!

Alkaline diet takes into account that your digestive system needs to be cleansed, but there are some additional steps you can take to speed up this process.

- **Digestive foods** – certain types of food can help you quickly detoxify your digestive system. These foods include avocado, greens, broccoli, celery, sweet potatoes, and chickpeas. When you feel like having a snack, go for grapefruit, which is mildly alkaline, and it contains pectin fiber, which is known as an excellent cleanser for the digestive system. On the other hand, make sure to avoid foods that are bad for you, such as trans -fats, processed foods, yeast, sugar, etc.
- **Digestive supplements** – you can use fiber supplements, such as psyllium husks. There are also other supplements that help your digestion, so make sure to check out for them in the local pharmacy or a drug store. The one thing you want to ensure is that they contain no sugar or artificial ingredients.
- **Stay hydrated** – once again, drinking enough fluids proves to be essential for your organism. Drinking enough water every day helps your digestive system and your entire body.
- **Take your time with chewing** – this is also known as premature swallowing, and it's caused by talking while eating and incomplete chewing. You see, the digestive system cannot digest big food chunks, so eating large pieces leads to digestive discomfort. The entire process of digestion actually starts in your mouth with chewing.

On top of that, digestive enzymes that get released through chewing are essential for the further digestion process.

- **Have enough time for a meal** – if you are under stress or in a rush to head out, you can properly eat, and that also stresses your digestive system. When you are eating, you need to take your time. Every meal should be a way of relaxing. You should also make sure not to reach for your fork until you completely chew and swallow your current mouthful. There is no reason not to savor every bite and enjoy your meal.

Eat Regularly and Avoid Big Meals

Large meals impose a lot of stress on your digestive system. That is why it's important to eat on a regular basis and to eat smaller or moderate meals. Normal eating will also prevent you from feeling hungry quickly after a meal and keep you from having an unhealthy acidic snack.

The point of this section is to prove that the way of eating is equally important as what you eat. I'm sure that you felt bloated or suffered problems after you just induced a significant amount of food in a matter of minutes. The simple tips to help your digestive system will assist you in improving the results of your diet through no extra work.

Don't Be Afraid to Eat

When people start a new diet, they think that the goal is to eat as little as they can. They believe that small meals will help them get rid of those extra pounds. Believe it or not, this is wrong!

Yes, there is such thing as consuming too much food, but there is absolutely no reason to be restricted to small meals. Furthermore, when it comes to alkaline diet, the best way to clean your body of acids is to load it with nutrients. And what better way to secure you induced enough healthy ingredients than eating a lot?

Believe it or not, the worst thing you can do on the alkaline diet is to have a plain salad as your meal. You need to make sure that you induce enough of various foods to secure all the required nutrients to make your body slightly alkaline. As long as you follow the ratio of 80/20 for alkaline foods, you are good. There is one thing to make sure on the alkaline diet – you shouldn't be hungry at any moment. Believe it or not, feeling hungry is an acidic state, so you need to make sure to avoid that from happening. If you are feeling hungry often, then you probably need to make some adjustments to your nutrition plan. Make sure not to miss any meals and vital nutrients that your body needs to work properly. Having three meals during the day is a must, and there is no reason not to throw in some healthy snacks, such as seeds or nuts, and even tomato or avocado.

Concerns About Alkaline Diet

We have previously established that the keyword in the alkaline diet is a balance. The ideal pH level throughout your body should be between 7.2 and 7.4, which is actually a slightly alkaline state for your organism. While it's not good to have an overly acidic body, it's equally wrong to reach a high level of alkalinity. That state is also known as alkalosis, and it occurs when you have excess alkali or base in your body.

You can get too alkaline if you have higher bicarbonate or lower carbon dioxide levels. The first one is also called metabolic alkalosis, while the other is known as respiratory alkalosis. You can also suffer from hypokalemic alkalosis (extreme lack of potassium) and hypochloremic alkalosis (severe lack of chloride).

Symptoms of Alkalosis

There are certain symptoms you can notice that might be related to alkalosis. The first one is confusion, which is dangerous because it can lead to fainting or even coma. You might also feel hand tremor, prolonged muscle spasms or muscle twitching. Numbness in your arms, legs, and face, as well as tingling, are also symptoms that can occur during alkalosis. You can also feel nausea and even start vomiting, or you can be unable to catch your breath. You can try to help your breathing by using a paper bag to breathe into it. Aside from that, the best way to correct the imbalance caused by alkalosis is to take medications, so make sure to call your health provider if you experience any of the symptoms.

Hypokalemia

Alkalosis can cause hypokalemia, which is nothing else than extreme lack of potassium in your body. Potassium is crucial for our organism to properly conduct various processes, such as proper cell function, including muscle and nerve cells. Aside from eating and metabolic disorders, medications can cause hypokalemia. You should avoid chewing tobacco that contains glycyrrhetinic acid, as well as drinking a lot of herbal teas and eating a lot of licorice. Symptoms of hypokalemia include fatigue, constipation, and paralysis of vital body organs.

Arrhythmias

Heart arrhythmias can occur if you reach alkalosis. In case you don't know, the arrhythmia is irregular heart beat (it can be both too slow and too fast). Symptoms of arrhythmia include chest pain, heart palpitations, fainting, and shortness of breath. You may notice that you are sweating more than usual and that your skin became pale. If not taken care of, arrhythmias may lead to heart failure, heart attack, or a stroke that can even be fatal.

Coma

If your blood has excessive alkaline levels, you may go into a coma, which is a deep and profound state of unconsciousness. Comas can last up to three or four weeks (rarely longer), and you can completely recover when it comes to awareness. However, more often than not, people that wake up from a coma suffer intellectual, physical or psychological problems. In some cases, people don't recover their awareness completely, and they stay in a partially vegetative state. That is why you should be especially careful not to have excessive alkalosis levels in your body.

Chapter 6:
Breakfast Recipes

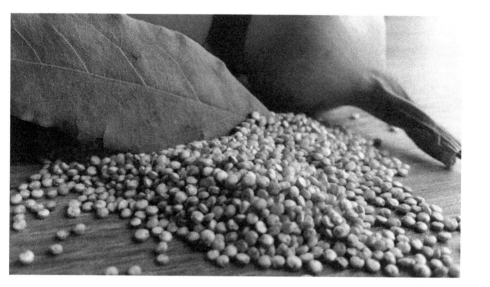

Quinoa Porridge
Prep time: 6 minutes

Cook time: 7 minutes

Serves 2

Ingredients

- 1 vanilla essence
- ½ lemon zest, grated
- ½ cup coconut milk (alternatively, you can use coconut cream)
- ½ teaspoon ground nutmeg
- ½ teaspoon of cinnamon (or 1 stick)
- 1 cup organic quinoa, dry
- 1 ½ teaspoons ground ginger
- 1 teaspoon ground cloves
- 2 cups of alkaline water (or pure)
- A handful of nuts and seeds for garnish

Directions

Check the package instructions and prepare the quinoa in accordance with them. Make sure that you drain it after cooking.

Use a saucepan and add drained quinoa to it. Also add ground cloves, ground nutmeg, ground ginger, and cinnamon. Stir the ingredients well to combine.

Add coconut milk (or cream) and vanilla essence. Stir everything to combine the ingredients. Once you heat everything and properly combine the ingredients, transfer them to a serving bowl.

Sprinkle with a handful of nuts and seeds of your choice and garnish. You can drink coconut yogurt with quinoa porridge.

Carrot and Hemp Seed Muffins
Prep time: 5 minutes

Cook time: 25 minutes

Serves 4

Ingredients:

- 3 tablespoons water
- 1 tablespoon ground flaxseed
- 2 cups oat flour
- 1 cup almond milk (boxed)
- ½ cup unrefined whole cane sugar, such as Sucanat
- 1 carrot, shredded
- 6 tablespoons cashew butter
- 2 tablespoons hemp seeds
- 1 tablespoon chopped lacinato kale
- 1 tablespoon baking powder
- ⅛ teaspoon vanilla bean powder
- Pinch sea salt

Directions

Preheat the oven to 350°F.

To prepare a flax egg, in a small bowl, whisk together the water and flaxseed.

Transfer the flax egg to a medium bowl, and add the oat flour, almond milk, sugar, carrot, cashew butter, hemp seeds, kale, baking powder, vanilla bean powder, and salt, stirring until well combined.

Divide the mixture evenly among 12 muffin cups, bake for 20 to 25 minutes, and enjoy right away.

Turmeric Tofu Scramble
Prep time: 5 minutes

Cook time: 10 minutes

Servings: 2

Ingredients:

- 8 ounces firm tofu
- ¼ teaspoon salt, see notes
- ¼ teaspoon turmeric powder, see notes
- 1/8 teaspoon ground black pepper

Directions

Squeeze and drain the liquid out of the tofu.

Chop it finely, then crumble it using a fork.

Heat some oil in the pan and stir in tofu along with other ingredients.

Stir cook for 10 minutes.

Garnish with parsley.

Serve and enjoy.

Good Morning Popeye
Prep time: 5 minutes

Cook time: 10 minutes

Serves 2

Ingredients:

- 1 Tbsp coconut oil
- 2 medium sweet potatoes, peeled and cubed
- 1 medium sweet onion, chopped
- 1 red bell pepper, seeded, chopped
- ¼ cup sliced mushrooms, any type
- 2 garlic cloves, chopped
- 4 cups spinach
- 1 tsp onion powder
- 1 tsp garlic powder
- ½ tsp dried herbs such as rosemary or sage
- ½ tsp sea salt

Directions

In a medium bowl, combine the oil, sweet potatoes, onion, red bell pepper, mushrooms, garlic, spinach, onion powder, garlic powder, dried herb, and salt.

Toss the vegetables in the oil until evenly coated.

Heat a nonstick frying pan over medium heat and cook the vegetables, stirring, for 10 minutes, or until tender.

Divide into two portions and serve.

Alkaline Muesli
Prep time: 6 minutes

Serves 1

Ingredients:

- 1 cup coconut milk, unsweetened (you can use almond milk instead)
- 1 tablespoon almonds, sliced
- ½ cup apple, chopped
- ½ cup rolled oats, gluten-free
- A dash of cinnamon

Directions

Use a serving bowl and add unsweetened coconut milk and rolled oats in it. Cut the apples and slice the almonds and throw them into the mixture, as well as a dash of cinnamon. Combine everything if to mix the ingredients.

Place the oats in the fridge for at least an hour to soak (you can also soak them the night before).

Chapter 7:
Juices and Smoothies

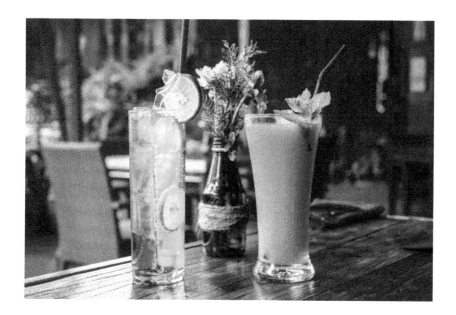

Avocado Paradise
Prep time: 5 minutes

Serves 2

Ingredients:

- ½ avocado, cubed
- 1 cup coconut milk
- Half a lemon
- ¼ cup fresh spinach leaves
- 1 pear
- 1 tablespoon hemp. Seed powder

Directions

Blend all the ingredients until smooth

Add a few ice cubes to make it chilled

Add your desired toppings

Enjoy!

Mango and Lime Smoothie
Prep time: 6 minutes

Serves 2

Ingredients:

- 2 tablespoon lime juice
- 2 cups spinach, chopped and stemmed
- 1½ cups frozen mango, cubed
- 1 cup green grapes

Directions

Add the listed ingredients to your blender and blend until smooth

Serve chilled!

Almond Coconut Smoothie
Prep time: 5 minutes

Serves 1

Ingredients:

- 2 cups skimmed milk
- 3 tablespoons Pip + Nut Coconut Almond butter
- 2 bananas
- 1 tablespoon flax seeds
- 2 teaspoons old fashioned oats
- 1 tablespoon honey

Directions

Add all the ingredients to a blender.

Blend well until smooth.

Refrigerate for 2 to 3 hours.

Serve.

Apple Almond Smoothie
Prep time: 5 minutes

Serves 1

Ingredients:

- 1 cup apple cider
- ½ cup coconut yogurt
- 4 tablespoons almonds, crushed
- ¼ teaspoon cinnamon
- ¼ teaspoon nutmeg
- 1 cup ice cubes

Directions

Add all the ingredients to a blender.

Blend well until smooth.

Serve.

Banana Blend
Prep time: 4 minutes

Serves 1

Ingredients:

- 2 bananas
- Ice cubes

Directions

Blend until smooth and then serve.

Chapter 8:
Soups

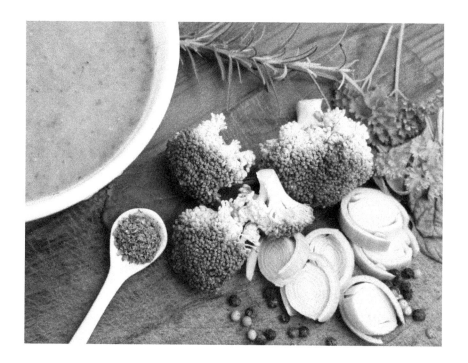

Cucumber and Lime Soup
Prep time: 6 minutes

Serves 1 or 2

Ingredients:

- 1 cucumber, peeled
- ½ zucchini, peeled
- 1 tablespoon freshly squeezed lime juice
- 1 tablespoon fresh cilantro leaves
- 1 garlic clove, crushed
- ¼ teaspoon sea salt

Directions

In a blender, blend together the cucumber, zucchini, lime juice, cilantro, garlic, and salt until well combined. Add more salt, if necessary.

Pour into 1 large or 2 small bowls and enjoy immediately, or refrigerate for 15 to 20 minutes to chill before serving.

Vegetable Soup
Prep time: 7 minutes

Serves 2

Ingredients:

- 2 cups carrots, chopped
- ½ cup fresh peas
- 1 tablespoon shallot chopped
- ½ inch piece of ginger
- 2 cups water
- ½ large avocado
- ½ teaspoon Celtic sea salt
- A drizzle of hazelnut oil, for garnish
- Chopped cilantro, for garnish

Directions

Add everything to a blender except the garnishes.

Process the ingredients at low speed.

Adjust seasoning with the spices.

Garnish with cilantro and hazelnut oil.

Serve.

BBB Soup
Prep time: 4 minutes

Cook time: 10 minutes

Serves: 2

Ingredients:

- 3 cups vegetable broth
- 1 cup bok choy, chopped
- 1 bunch broccolini, chopped roughly
- ½ cup brown rice, cooked
- 2-3 carrots, peeled, sliced

Directions

In a saucepan over medium heat, combine all ingredients.

Bring to a simmer and cook for 10 minutes, or until the vegetables are cooked and tender. Serve.

Carrot Sweet Potato Soup
Prep time: 6 minutes

Cook time: 30 minutes

Serves 4

Ingredients:

- 1 tablespoon coconut oil
- 2 cups yellow onion, chopped
- 2 cloves garlic, minced
- 1 tablespoon fresh ginger, minced
- 2 tablespoons red curry paste
- 4 cups low-sodium vegetable broth
- 3 cups diced carrots, peeled
- 3 cups sweet potatoes, peeled and diced
- Celtic sea salt, iodine free, to taste
- Freshly ground black pepper to taste
- ¼ teaspoon cayenne pepper

Directions

Sauté garlic, onion, and ginger in a greased pan for 5 to 6 minutes.

Stir in curry paste and broth.

Mix well then add carrots, salt, and sweet potatoes

Boil the soup on high heat. Cover the pot. Cook for 15 to 20 minutes.

Blend this soup in a blender in batches until smooth.

Adjust seasoning with salt and pepper.

Divide the soup into the serving bowl.

Serve warm.

Kale Soup
Prep time: 5 minutes

Cook time: 30 minutes

Serves: 2

Ingredients:

- 1 small onion, chopped
- 3 cloves garlic, minced
- 2 celery stalks, diced
- 2 tablespoons red wine
- 4 tablespoons olive oil or coconut oil
- 4 cups vegetable stock
- 1 teaspoon Himalayan salt
- ¼ teaspoon black pepper
- ¼ teaspoon dried basil (or 1 tsp fresh)
- 1 can cooked chickpeas, rinsed and drained
- 1 cup kale no stems, ale, cut into strips

Directions

First, sauté celery, garlic and onion in the oil for 3-4 minutes (medium heat)

Add veggie stock as well as basil, chickpeas, salt and pepper.

Bring to a boil (covered). Reduce heat and simmer for about 15 minutes on medium heat.

Blend the mixture.

Once blended, pour the mixture back into the pot, adding the kale and simmering for 10 minutes. Serve hot.

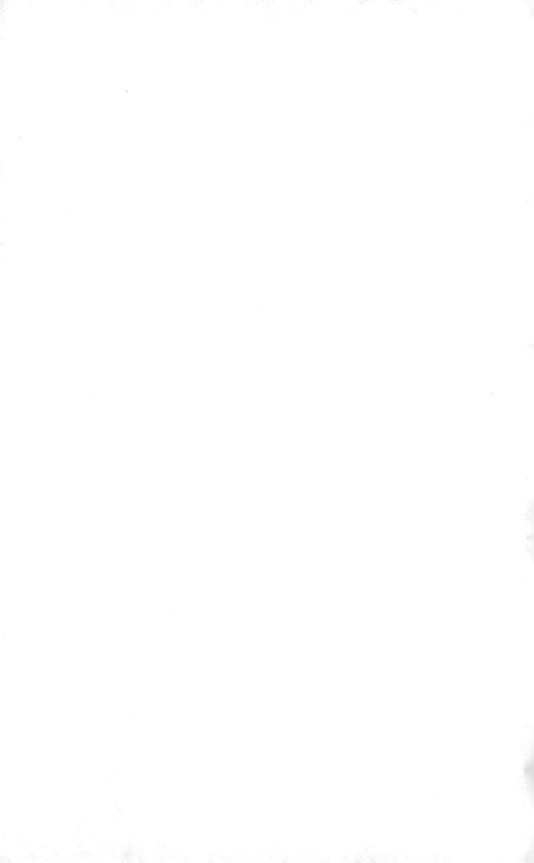

CPSIA information can be obtained
at www.ICGtesting.com
Printed in the USA
BVHW090943280121
598991BV00005B/329